Contents

INTRODUCTION

For thousands of years medicine men and 'wise women' have known that herbs possess remarkable healing properties. Today, empirical evidence gathered over the centuries is being backed-up by scientific studies: ancient wisdom is meeting the data of the white-coated lab technician. In addition, herbs from all over the world is now easily available, and at Indigo Herbs you'll find them cost-effective too.

There are many herbs to support men's health, and unlike synthetic pharmaceutical drugs, they rarely have side-effects. Whether you want to relieve stress, boost your sexual drive, sharpen your mental faculties, or increase your physical resilience for training, there is a herb to fit the bill.

Although herbs can work wonders on their own, they function most effectively when used as part of a healthy lifestyle – a balanced wholefood diet, detoxification, regular exercise, relaxation, ade□uate sleep, and emotional/spiritual fulfilment.

Today's man wants to take responsibility for his health and a good place to start is nutrition. Superfoods are nutrient-dense plants such as berries, seeds, algae, mushrooms, seaweeds and grasses. Used as a daily supplement, added to juices or smoothies, sprinkled on yoghurt or cereal, or made into raw-food energy bars (go on, experiment!), they can □uickly transform your diet from 2-star to 5-star.

CHAPTER ONE

HERBS FOR MEN

hawthorn (Crataegus oxyacantha and C. monogyna)

Parts used: Leaves, flowers, berries, and tips of branches

Benefits: Hawthorn may well be the herb supreme for the heart, and a healthy heart is essential to a long and productive life. The flowers, berries, tips of branches, and leaves nourish, strengthen, and tone the heart muscle and its blood vessels. As a tonic for the heart, it has the amazing ability to either gently stimulate or depress the heart's activity as needed. Hawthorn dilates arteries and veins, allowing blood to flow more freely and releasing cardiovascular constrictions and blockages. It lowers blood pressure and also helps maintain healthy cholesterol levels. Hawthorn is outstanding both for preventing heart problems and for treating heart disease, edema, angina, and heart arrhythmia. Because of its strong concentrations of bioflavonoids, hawthorn is an effective antioxidant and is used to fight free radicals in the system. Though it is little is mentioned in literature, hawthorn is also a wonderful remedy for "broken hearts" and for depression and anxiety. It is a specific medicine for those who have a difficult time expressing their feelings or who suppress their emotions. Hawthorn helps the heart flower, open, and be healed.

The hawthorn tree has been planted in or near most herb gardens throughout Europe and has been revered and surrounded by legend for centuries. When my grandmother came to thiscountry, she planted hawthorns in the yard of each home she lived in. Many of those old hawthorns planted by her strong, worn hands still bloom.

Suggested uses: Hawthorn is a tonic herb and should be used over a period of time to be effective. Use in the form of tea, tincture, capsules, syrup, and jam or jelly. The general dose would be 3 to 4 cups of tea a day, 1 teaspoon of the tincture three times daily, or 2 capsules three times daily. However, hawthorn tastes so good and is generally recommended more culinary-style preparations, such as jam, jelly, and liqueur, which taste exquisite and retain all of the herb's nourishing benefits. Hawthorn berry jam, in particular, is delicious and readily available in grocery stores, as well as pharmacies. Spread it on crackers and consume to your heart's delight. Hawthorn berries also make a delicious tea and are often combined with lemon balm and oats for hypertension. Another treatment for high blood pressure is a tea made of hawthorn leaves, berries, or flowers combined with yarrow and motherwort. Hawthorn berries, leaves, and flowers are also excellent combined with ginkgo leaves as a vascular tonic.

Damiana (Turnera aphrodisiaca)

Parts used: Leaves

Benefits: Though damiana has a strong reputation as an herb of passion and romance, It is included in a list of favorite longevity herbs because it is completely restorative; it restores exhausted nerves, exhausted dreams, and exhausted spirit. It will help restore sexual vitality; its species name, aphrodisiaca, is a sure giveaway. Damiana has long been known to strengthen the reproductive systems of both men and women. Its nervine and toning properties make damiana a good general herb for the nervous system, as well, and as a relaxant and antidepressant. It is also a favorite herb to use for dream work. It stimulates and promotes one's ability to remember dreams and often will promote colorful, though not always positive, dreamlike states.

Suggested uses: Use in cases of diminished sexual vitality, impotence, infertility, nervous exhaustion, anxiety and depression associated with sexual factors, and muscle and nerve exhaustion, as well as for dream therapy. Damiana is most often administered in tincture or capsule form. It is also very effective as tea but should be blended with other, more tasty herbs, such as oats and lemon balm, because of its bitter flavor.

Turmeric

This is one of the best herbs for immune health and is often overlooked because of the huge popularity of echinacea. But it has upheld its reputation for its immune-enhancing properties for centuries and is highly regarded for its antitumor and antibiotic activities. In East Indian medicine, it is valued as a blood purifier and metabolic tonic. It is used to reduce fevers, improve poor circulation, and relieve skin disorders. It is highly valued as a first-aid item for boils, burns, sprains, swelling, and bruises.

Astragalus (Astragalus membranaceus)

Traditionally prescribed in Chinese Medicine for male infertility, Astragalus has now been scientifically proven to increase sperm motility in a study conducted by the Institutes of Traditional Medicine and Clinical Medicine. It is extremely supportive of male hormones, by balancing glucose levels it can optimise testosterone and growth hormone levels.

It is a powerful immune booster, with the ability to stimulate the body's NK (natural killer) cells and increasing the production of "interferon", which helps to improve resistance to viral infections. Astragalus also slows down the aging process and revitalises the entire body, by stimulating the production of stem cells in the bone marrow.

Catuaba Bark (Erythroxylum catuaba)

The name Catuaba is a Guarani word that translates as "what gives strength to the Indian". It is the most famed and sought after aphrodisiac, with numerous songs composed by the Tupi Indians in praise of its libido enhancing effects and ability to treat erectile dysfunction. Research shows that Catuaba bark may enhance erectile strength by widening blood vessels, allowing more blood to flow to the penis. Also known as Brazilian Viagra, Catuaba contains "yohimbine", thought to be the active compound that provides a stimulatory effect to the libido.

It is also used as an overall energy booster, for stimulating the nervous system, sharpening memory and focus and to combat fatigue.

Gokshura (Tribulus terrestris)

Gokshura (Tribulus Terrestris) is rich in "saponins" – phytochemicals that have the ability to increase the body's testosterone levels naturally. This makes it a great herb for bodybuilding, training and a powerful sexual tonic.

As an aphrodisiac, Gokshura tops the charts of herbal Viagra. Studies have shown that Gokshura elevates the luteinising hormone (LH), increasing the levels of free testosterone in healthy males. This in turn will increase sexual desire and libido, improve the □uality of sperm whilst making it more nimble, in some cases it will help to remedy erectile dysfunction and it has been proven to be helpful in cases of premature ejaculation. This herb will stimulate the production of sex hormones without affecting other bodily systems.

Gokshura truly shines as a bodybuilding or training supplement. Of the aforementioned saponins, it contains one steroidal saponin in particular – protodioscin – which is thought to be the active nutrient responsible for this herb's popularity amongst athletes. This muscle building compound is also renowned for increasing strength and enhancing athletic performance.

Other health benefits men can expect from this versatile herb include; restorative sleep, positive mood, pain reduction and protection of the cardiovascular system.

Horny Goat Weed (Epimedium sagittatum)

Behind its comical name, Horny Goat Weed stands as a time tested aphrodisiac that increases libido in both men and women and improves erectile function in men. This is thought to be due, in part, to the flavonoid "icariin", which is also responsible for the best known health benefits associated with this herb.

Firstly, icariin has been found to have the ability to boost the successful transmission of Nitric Oxide, the primary chemical transmitter for the successful and ample delivery of blood delivery to the penis tissue. Secondly it increases the natural circulation of free form testosterone around the body, not only boosting libido – testosterone is crucial to the health of the prostate and plays a dominant role in the production of healthy sperm. Horny Goat Weed can also benefit men in the gym, increasing lean muscle mass, improving muscular "pump" and enhancing levels of stamina and endurance.

Mucuna / Kapikachhu (Mucuna pruriens)

Researchers at the Department of Biochemistry, Chhatrapati Medical University in India found that Kapikachhu supports the normal function of the male reproductive system, in particular supporting normal levels of male fertility. This appears to be related to the ability of this herb to; increase libido (men and women), increase sperm count, enhance blood circulation to the genitals, strengthen and tone the sexual glands and release bound up testosterone – increasing the level of bio-available testosterone.

Kapikachhu is also especially beneficial to brain health, its primary compound "levadopa" (L-dopa) is a precursor to dopamine, adrenaline and noradrenaline. Whilst dopamine is most commonly associated with pleasure, it actually plays a critical role in muscle control. L-dopa is synthesized in the brain into dopamine, and is often used as a treatment in Parkinson's disease. By raising low dopamine levels, Kapikachhu can have a positive effect on motivation, attention span, the ability to relax and general mental well-being.

Muira Puama (Ptychopetalum)

Also known as "potency wood", Muira Puama has long been used by the Amazonian people to manage a variety of age related conditions. It is marketed in Brazil as a "body stimulant, energetic tonic and aphrodisiac". It can be especially useful in supporting healthy erectile response and restoring libido in men suffering the effects of fatigue or age related complaints.

Muira Puama contains "sterols", the building blocks of sex hormones such as testosterone. One study found that this herb relaxes the corpus cavernosa – a sponge like area that holds blood during an erection. This relaxation allows more blood to flow to the penis, producing a stronger and firmer erectile response. Dr Jacques Maynberg conducted two studies at the Institute of Sexology in Paris, where he gave men stricken with low libido and diminished erectile capacity Muira Puama for two weeks. In both studies between 60% - 70% of the men reported a notable increase in libido and an improvement in their ability to maintain an erection.

In addition to its aphrodisiac ualities, Muira Puama has been used for stress management, nervous system stimulation and as a general overall health tonic.

Pumpkin Seed Protein (Cucurbita pepo)

Aside from providing a good serving of high □uality, complete, plant based protein, Pumpkin Seed Protein Powder can have a beneficial effect on the health of the prostate. Benign Prostate Hyperplasia (or enlargement of the prostrate gland) is common in men over 50 years of age. Over stimulation of the prostate cells is caused by the hormone dihydrotestosterone (DHT). The phytosterols found in pumpkin seeds have been found to inhibit the production of DHT, leading to a decrease in the uncomfortable symptoms associated with BPH.

Pumpkin Seed Protein Powder is also high in zinc – an essential mineral in the treatment of BPH.

Tongkat Ali (Eurycoma longifolia)

Testosterone and other male hormones are known to decrease with age which can result in a condition known as "andropause" (also known as the male menopause). Symptoms can include lack of energy, a decrease in libido, increased body fat and mental lethargy. Tongkat Ali is a powerful herb that has been traditionally used for centuries as a remedy for age-related male disorders. Many studies show that this root contains compounds that stimulate libido, promote sperm motility and semen quality and support muscle growth - all effects that are attributed to an increase in testosterone. The hormonal support provided by

Tongkat Ali can also increase male fertility by promoting normal sperm quality.

This effect is backed up by a 2012 study of 76 men, only 35 percent of whom had normal testosterone levels. After one month of supplementation with Tongkat Ali, the number of men with normal testosterone levels had risen significantly to 90 percent. Another pleasant side effect of this increase in testosterone is a boost in sex drive, with it long being used in South East Asia as an aphrodisiac.

Nettle (Urtica dioica)

Parts used: Leaves, seeds, roots, and young tops

Benefits: This is the stinging nettle that farmers despise, hikers hate, and children learn to avoid.

But herbalists around the world fall at the feet of this green goddess/green man herb. It is one of the superior tonic herbs and is as important as many of the famous Chinese "long life" herbs. It is a vitamin factory, rich in iron, calcium, potassium, silicon, magnesium, manganese, zinc, and chromium, as well as a host of other vitamins and minerals. One favorite all-around remedies, it makes a great hair and scalp tonic. It activates themetabolism by strengthening and toning the entire system. It is useful for growing pains in young children, when their bones and joints ache. An excellent reproductive tonic for men and women, nettle is used for alleviating the symptoms of PMS and menopause. It's a superb herb for the genitourinary system and will strengthen weak kidneys, essential for vitality and energy. It is indicated for liver problems and is excellent for allergies and hay fever.

Valerian (Valeriana officinalis)

Parts used: Roots

Benefits: Valerian has been highly regarded as an herbal medicine for centuries. Hildegard von Bingen, a famous 12th-century German abbess and herbalist, valued it as a sedative. In the 1500s, the great herbalist Gerard claimed that valerian was one of the most popular remedies of his time. Today, in spite of its distinct and somewhat offensive odor, valerian continues to be one of the most popular medicinal herbs in the world.

There is no finer herb than valerian for those who suffer from stress, insomnia, and nervous system disorders; it is powerful, safe, very effective, and nonaddictive. Its name is derived from the Latin valere, "to be well" or "to be strong." In Europe, where it has been used for centuries, valerian can be found in hundreds of over-the-counter drugs and is relied on primarily as a medicine for stress and tension. It is effective for insomnia, pain, restlessness, headaches, digestive problems due to nerves, and muscle spasms. Depending on the individual, the smell is either relished or deemed offensive. Rather love the odor, which reminds people of violets, rich sweet earth, or dirty underwear, depending on the age of the root.

Valerian is effective both as a long-term nerve tonic and as a remedy for acute problems such as headaches and pain. It has powerful tonic effects on the heart and is often recommended in combination with hawthorn berries for high blood pressure and irregular heartbeat.

Suggested uses: Because the root is rich in volatile oils, it should be infused rather than decocted. Valerian is often tinctured or encapsulated rather than taken as tea because of its odor, though its taste is quite pleasant. Herbalists are in disagreement about whether the fresh or dried herb works better. Without a doubt, it's better tasting when fresh. Cats love it, often better than catnip.

Caution: Valerian is generally considered a safe, nontoxic herb. It is used as a relaxant, but it can have the opposite effect on people who are particularly sensitive to it. If you become further agitated and restless after taking valerian, discontinue use and consider yourself in that rare 5 percent of the population that cannot tolerate this herb.

Saw Palmetto (Serenoa repens)

Parts used: Berries

Benefits: Though long used by the native people of the subtropical coast of North America, saw palmetto has risen rapidly in popularity in recent years. It is simply the best remedy for inflammation of the prostate gland. It is tonic in action and serves as an effective diuretic and relaxant. It is strengthening to those individuals who are continuously nervous and stressed and who lack energy and vitality. Its fatty fruit is one of the few Western herbs that are anabolic; it encourages weight gain and bulk by strengthening and building body tissue. It is used by womento firm sagging breast tissue. As a tonic herb, it can be taken on a regular basis to strengthen the urinary and endocrine systems and to prevent future problems with the prostate gland. Why wait?

Nicknamed the "plant catheter," saw palmetto has the ability to strengthen the neck of the bladder and to reduce enlarged prostate glands. It reduces many of the problems associated with an enlarged prostate gland: dribbling urine; slow, painful urination; the need to urinate several times during the night; and incomplete urination, which can lead to low-grade cystitis.

Suggested uses: Saw palmetto has a fatty, pungent flavor that is hard to swallow and hard to disguise. It is difficult to conceive of the taste of this herb until you've tried it. Not many know of many people who enjoy its flavor in tea. It's usually available in tincture form. It can be used in capsules as well, but they should be fresh and of good quality, because the fats in saw palmetto quickly turn rancid.

Ashwagandha (Withania somnifera)

Parts used: Roots

Benefits: An ancient Ayurvedic herb, ashwagandha is often referred to as the "Indian ginseng," and, in fact, it is used in very much the same manner that ginseng is used in Asia. An excellent adaptogenic herb, ashwagandha increases the body's overall ability to adapt to and resist stress.

In India, it is used to increase memory and facilitate learning. It is both energizing and soothing. Ashwagandha is primarily classified as a male tonic herb, but women use it as well. It is a classic reproductive tonic and will help restore sexual chi, or energy.

Suggested uses: This herb is specifically indicated for reduced levels of energy, general debilitation, reduced sexual energy, nervous tension, stress, and anxiety. It promotes general well-being and enhances stamina (thus explaining its popularity with athletes). Said to have the smell of a female horse's urine and the stamina of a stallion, ashwagandha isn't the best-tasting herb you'll ever meet. Blend it with other more flavorful herbs, such as ginger, sarsaparilla, and cinnamon, to make a suitable-tasting tea. Powder the root and mix it with milk for a classic Indian rejuvenating drink, or try blending it with your favorite chai tea blend. You can also use it in tincture or capsule form.

Yarrow (Achillea millefolium)

Parts used: Leaves and flowers

Benefits: A beautiful roadside weed, yarrow is best recognized by its creamy flowers, which bloom throughout the summer months. It is an excellent diaphoretic, often used in teas to promote sweating, thereby helping reduce fevers. Yarrow is a classic first-aid herb and can be used to stop bleeding both internally and externally. It is effective for both menstrual and stomach cramps and is often used in formulas for stomach flus. It also has beneficial effects for the heart and lungs.

Suggested uses: Yarrow makes a bitter infusion, so blend it with tastier herbs as a digestive aid and diaphoretic. The dried, powdered leaf is useful in a first-aid kit; it can be applied to cuts and wounds to disinfect and stop bleeding. A pinch of the powder can be placed in the nose to stop a nosebleed.

CHAPTER 2

RECIPES

Fertility & Potency Syrup

This formula has a reputation for increasing virility in men and helping with fertility (if not due to structural causes). It is a tonic formula and needs to be used over a period of 3 to 6 months.

1 ginseng root

2 ounces muira puama

1 ounce ashwagandha

½ ounce saw palmetto berries

½ ounce wild yam root

2 quarts water

2 ounces oats (milky green tops)

½ ounce raspberry leaf

1 ounce damiana

1 ounce nettles

1 to 2 cups honey (or to taste)

1 cup fruit concentrate (available in natural foods stores)

½ cup brandy (optional, but will help preserve syrup)

1. Combine the ginseng, muira puama, ashwagandha, saw palmetto berries, and wild yam with the water. Decoct slowly, as instructed, over low heat until the liquid has been reduced to 1 quart. Keep the lid slightly ajar so that some of the steam can evaporate.

2. Turn off the heat and immediately add the oats, raspberryleaf, damiana, and nettles. Cover tightly and let the herbs sit overnight.

3. The next day, strain the herbs through a finemesh strainer lined with muslin or cheesecloth. Add honey to taste, the fruitconcentrate, and the brandy. Store in the refrigerator. Take 2 to 4 tablespoons daily for 3 to 6 months.

Men's Long-Life Elixir

This is one of an all-time favorite recipe.

; this formula is predominantly a masculine yang type of tonic that builds strength and vitality.

2 parts damiana leaf

2 parts fo-ti

2 parts ginger root

2 parts licorice

2 parts sassafras root bark

2 parts wild yam root

1 part Chinese star anise

1 part sarsaparilla root

½ part saw palmetto berries

Asian ginseng roots (2 good-sized, □uality roots for each quart of tincture)

Brandy

Black cherry concentrate (available at most health food stores)

1. Prepare a tincture with the herbs and brandy, as instructed Let the mixture sit for 6 to 8 weeks; the longer, the better.

2. Strain. To each cup of liquid, add ½ cup of black cherry concentrate. Be sure this is a fruit concentrate, not a fruit juice. Shake well and rebottle. put the ginseng roots back into the rebottled tincture. A standard daily dose is about cup — just enough for an evening aperitif. Try sipping it with your sweetie before a sensuous night.

Energy Balls

This special, high-powered food supplement is delicious and easy to make. Though there are many "superfood bars" on the market, they are expensive and generally not as good as what you can make at home. Try these; they contain nutrients essential to the yang male energy system. They are energizing, restorative, and formulated to build and renew the male reproductive system when used over time. Be sure the herbs are finely powdered, or else you'll be picking out little chunks of nonchewable roots.

3 parts pumpkin seeds, powdered

2 parts Siberian ginseng powder

1 part ginkgo or gotu kola powder

1 part ginseng powder

½ part spirulina or Super Blue Green Algae

1 cup sesame butter (tahini)

½ cup honey

½ cup crushed almonds

Coconut, cocoa powder, raisins, chocolate or carob

chips, and granola for flavor

Carob powder or powdered milk

1. Combine the powdered herbs and spirulina and mix well.

2. Combine the sesame butter and honey, mixing to form a paste. If you want your Energy Balls to be sweeter, add more honey.

3. Add enough of the powdered herbs to thicken, then add the almonds and the flavoring additions. Thicken to the desired consistency with the carob powder or powdered

milk. Roll into walnut-sized balls. Eat two Energy Balls daily.

Once-A-Day Male Tonic

Herbal pastes can be spread on toast, licked from the spoon, or added to boiling water for instant tea. Stored in the refrigerator, the paste will last indefinitely. Here's one version of the recipe.

2 parts fo-ti powder

1 part astragalus powder

1 part ashwagandha powder

1 part cardamom powder

1 part cinnamon powder

1 part licorice root powder

1 part Siberian ginseng powder

½ part echinacea powder

¼ part ginger powder

Honey

Fruit concentrate

Mix all the herbs in a bowl. Add enough honey and fruit concentrate (blended according to your taste) to form a paste. Pure rose water also can be added for an exotic flavor. Be sure that the paste is moist enough. It will dry out a bit in the refrigerator, even when tightly closed. If it becomes too dry, moisten it with a little more fruit concentrate and honey.

Good-Life Wine

This aromatic herbal wine should be served as a tonic It can be taken in small dosages of ¼ cup daily to promote health and well-being.

4 astragalus roots

1 good-□uality medium-sized ginseng root

1 ounce ashwagandha root

1 ounce damiana leaf

1 ounce fo-ti

2 tablespoons cardamom seeds, crushed

2 tablespoons Chinese star anise

A couple of cloves (for flavor)

A pinch of ginger root (for flavor)

1 quart good-quality wine

1. Place the herbs in a widemouthed canning jar and pour the wine over the mixture. Cover and let sit for 3 to 4 weeks in a warm location.

2. Strain and rebottle the liquid into the original wine bottle. The ginseng root can be sliced and added back to the wine.

Ginseng Tonic Tea

1 large, well-aged ginseng root

Water

1. Place the root in the cooker and cover with water. Tie the cooker shut, then place it in another pan filled with water. Cook over low heat for 6 to 8 hours.

2. Strain, and drink all of the resulting li□uid. It is very potent, to say the least.

Male Toner Tea

A flavorful, well-balanced tea especially formulated for the male system,

3 parts sarsaparilla

3 parts sassafras

1 part burdock root

1 part cinnamon

1 part Siberian ginseng

1 part Asian or American ginseng

1 part licorice

1 part muira puama

1 part wild yam

¼ part ginger

¼ part orange peel

Prepare a decoction as directed. Drink 3 to 4 cups daily.

Chai Hombre

There are literally thousands of recipes for chai, a robust, spicy herbal blend originating in India, Nepal, and Tibet. Following is a chai blend especially formulated for men. It has some of the traditional chai herbs, but added are a number of herbs for male health. Serve it hot or chilled with frothy steamed milk.

6 slices fresh ginger root, grated

5 tablespoons black tea leaves

3 tablespoons cinnamon chips (or 1 stick broken into small pieces)

1 tablespoon sliced fo-ti

1 tablespoon sliced ginseng root

1 tablespoon sliced licorice root

2 teaspoons crushed cardamom

6 black peppercorns

4 whole cloves

6 cups water

Honey

Steamed milk (cow's, soy, or rice)

Nutmeg or cinnamon

1. Gently warm the herbs and the water in a covered saucepan for 10 to 15 minutes. Do not boil.

2. Strain the mixture into a warmed teapot and add honey to taste. Pour into a large cup, add a generous heap of steamed milk, and sprinkle with nutmeg or cinnamon.

Damiana Chocolate Love Liqueur

1 ounce damiana leaves (dried)

2 cups vodka or brandy

1½ cups spring-water

1 cup honey

Vanilla extract

Rose water

Chocolate syrup

Almond extract

1. Soak the damiana leaves in the vodka or brandy for 5 days.

Strain; reserve the liquid in a bottle.

2. Soak the alcohol-drenched leaves in the spring-water for 3 days. Strain and reserve the liquid.

3. Over low heat, gently warm the water extract and dissolve the honey in it. Remove the pan from the heat, then add the alcohol extract and stir well. Pour into a clean bottle and add a dash of vanilla and a touch of rose water for flavor. Let it mellow for 1 month or longer; it gets smoother with age.

4. To each cup of damiana liqueur, add ½ cup of chocolate syrup, 2 or 3 drops of almond extract, and a touch more of rose water.

Bath Blends

These three wonderful bath blends are formulated especially for men. To use them, first combine the herbs, then mix in the essential oil. Place a handful of the mixture in a cotton bag, nylon sock, or muslin bag and tie it onto the nozzle of the tub. Run very hot water into the tub for a few minutes, letting the water run over the herb bundle. Then release the bundle into the tub and adjust the temperature of the water to your liking. As an alternative, you can prepare an extrastrong herbal tea, strain it, and add it directly to the bathwater.

Refreshing/Stimulating Bath Blend

If you need to energize, use this invigorating blend.

2 parts peppermint

2 parts rosemary

6 to 8 drops pine essential oil

Deep Relaxation Bath

Try this bath whenever you need to unwind. The recipe makes enough for four to six baths.

2 parts chamomile

2 parts sage

1 part hops

1 part lavender

6 to 8 drops clary sage or lavender essential oil

Bath Blend For Sore Muscles

Sore muscles will benefit from soaking in this eucalyptus, sage, and pine blend. The recipe makes enough for two to four baths.

2 parts eucalyptus leaf

2 parts sage

6 to 8 drops pine or sage essential oil

Good Health For The Prostate

The prostate is getting a lot of press these days. It may even be the most talked-about male organ; it's certainly in the running for second place. Even so, many men are still not sure what the prostate does, why it's important, or even where it's located, until it starts aching or creating health problems.

A chestnut-shaped organ no larger than a walnut, the prostate is a part-muscular, part-glandular organ that is locatedbelow the bladder and next to the rectum. It surrounds the urethra, the tube that runs from the bladder to the tip of the penis. If the prostate becomes inflamed or engorged, it s□ueezes the urethra, and bladder infections, urinary incontinence, and kidney problems ensue. The prostate is also directly related to fertility, because it produces and secretes into the semen an alkaline, proteinlike fluid that is critical for sperm motility.

The causes of prostatitis (inflammation of the prostate) are varied, but most are directly related to stress. Often, though not always, the stress may be of a sexual nature. Irregular sexual patterns, that is, intense sexual activity after a long period of inactivity or a period of inactivity after intense sexual play, can also be a precursor of prostatitis. It seems the prostate prefers regularity. Other factors that can contribute to prostatitis include an unhealthy diet, consumption of alcohol, consumption of caffeine-rich products, lack of physical exercise, too much sitting, infections of the gums and tonsils, and venereal disease.

The symptoms of prostatitis and BPH are similar. They include:

• Painful urination

• Difficulty in emptying the bladder completely

• Having to get up at night to urinate

• Reduced force when urinating

• Pain upon sitting

• Unexplained chills and fever

• Blood in the urine (sometimes)

Prostate problems generally respond incredibly well to home treatment, which includes lifestyle changes, dietary changes, and herbal remedies. However, if your symptoms don't improve within a few days of beginning treatment, you'll want to consult your holistic health care practitioner or physician for further examination and advice.

Dietary Treatments for the Prostate

Eat simple, nourishing foods to enhance prostate health, as well as overall health. Diet should consist primarily of steamed vegetables, grains, and miso or chicken soup. Add medicinal herbs such as echinacea, astragalus, fo-ti, and ginseng to the soup base. Include lemon juice and unsweetened cranberry juice in your daily diet. Don't eat foods that you know will further irritate the prostate gland. Caffeine-rich foods, alcohol, and sugar seem to be particularly irritating.

Several foods, vitamins, and minerals are excellent in helping alleviate prostate enlargement and inflammation, including:

• Pumpkin seeds (¼ to ½ cup or more daily)

• Cucumbers (2 to 3 daily)

• Calcium/magnesium (600 mg combined daily)

• Vitamin E (400 I.U. daily)

• Zinc (20 to 50 mg daily)

Watermelon Cooling Tonic

Watermelon seeds are a wonderful remedy for prostate imbalances. If watermelon is in season, you're in luck. Put as much watermelon and seeds as you can drink in one serving into a blender (cut off the rind). Add a handful of unsalted pumpkin seeds. Blend until creamy. Drink 1 Quart daily. Fresh watermelon is wonderful for the kidneys and the prostate, providing a mineral-rich flush. If there is a lot of congestion in the gland, this is an excellent cooling tonic.

If watermelon is not in season, you can still make this remedy by using the seeds of the watermelon. Watermelon seeds can be purchased at some herb stores, but why not collect and dry your own in the warm summer months? Place the watermelon seeds and the pumpkin seeds in the blender with unsweetened cranberry juice. Blend until creamy. Drink 3 to 4 cups daily.

Medicinal Teas for Prostatitis

The following two medicinal formulas are excellent remedies for swollen, inflamed prostate. Drink 3 to 4 cups daily of one or both formulas. For greater effect, add 10 drops of saw palmetto tincture and 10 drops of pygeum tincture to the tea.

PROSTATE FORMULA #1

This formula aids in better urinary flow.

3 parts corn silk

3 parts watermelon seeds

2 parts nettle

1 part cleavers

1 part uva-ursi

Infuse the herbs as instructed

PROSTATE FORMULA #2

This formula is designed to ease inflammation and congestion of the prostate.

2 parts marsh mallow root

1 part echinacea

1 part gravel root

1 part organically cultivated pygeum

1 part saw palmetto

Prepare as a tincture as instructed.

Making an Herbal Poultice

Though messy, poultices are very helpful for relieving congestion of the prostate. Mix equal amounts of clay, comfrey leaf, and slippery elm powder in a bowl with warm water. Place the mixture on gauze or muslin fabric and apply directly to the skin covering the gland twice a day for 20 minutes. Use a jockstrap or underwear to hold the poultice in place. You can also mix fresh comfrey leaves in a blender with a little water to make a paste, place the mixture on gauze or muslin fabric, and use this as a poultice. If nothing else is available, try an oatmeal poultice.

Hot and Cold Compresses

Hot and cold compresses are also very effective for relieving congestion of the prostate. This treatment re□uires a bit of willpower. Wrap an ice pack in a towel and place it directly on the skin covering the prostate. Leave it on for a minute or two. Remove the cold pack and place a hot compress on the skin for a few minutes. Repeat this process three or four times at least once a day.

Glandular imbalances

Lack of energy, depression, impotence, and lack of vitality characterize glandular imbalances. The usual route to resolve these problems is to seek □uick-fix stimulants such as caffeine to maintain energy, but these will only further exhaust already depleted energy levels. Instead, try some of the following suggestions to build and stabilize inner chi and vitality:

• Take Men's Long-Life Elixir daily.

• Eat two Energy Balls daily.

• Snack on organic pumpkin seeds.

• Drink 3 to 4 cups of Male Toner Tea daily .

• Eat a small piece of ginseng root daily, drink ginseng tea,

or take 2 ginseng capsules three times daily.

• Take a cold shower at least every other day

Impotence And Infertility

Infertility is the inability to conceive after a period of adequate effort (a one-year period, by clinical standards). The latest statistics show that men's systems are the root of at least 40 percent of couples' infertility problems. Most cases of male infertility are due to low sperm count and/or weak or inactive sperm. Stress and lack of activity can be contributing factors. Some less common causes are obstructions in the reproductive system, liver problems, and glandular imbalances in the thyroid (hypothyroidism) or the pituitary gland.

How Can Impotence and Infertility Be Treated?

Emphasize the following herbs in your formulas: Siberian ginseng, muira puama, saw palmetto, astragalus, ashwagandha, nettles, oats, dandelion, sarsaparilla, licorice, wild yam, and fo-ti, or ho shou wu.

• Follow the suggestions listed for prostate health, including use of saw palmetto.

• Take 400 I.U. of vitamin E daily.

• Take zinc supplements (30 ml) daily.

• Take 1 teaspoon of bee pollen daily.

• Establish a nonstressful but vigorous daily physical exercise program.

• Eat plenty of fresh raw vegetables, high-quality protein sources, fresh fruit, and grains. Avoid all processed refined foods, alcohol, sugar, and caffeine-rich foods.

• Every day, take 2 Energy Balls , ¼ cup of Men's Long-Life Elixir and 1 to 2 teaspoons of Once-a-Day Male Tonic

Genitourinary Infections

Though women tend to be more susceptible than men to urinary tract infections, men do experience many systemic imbalances as infections in their genitourinary system.

Inflamed Penis or Foreskin Infection

An infected foreskin can be painfully disruptive. There are several external applications that will cure an inflamed penis or infected foreskin.

• Herbal powder. The quickest and most effective action is to make a powder of 3 parts slippery elm powder or marsh mallow root powder to 1 part organically grown goldenseal powder. Sprinkle this powder over the head and shaft of the penis.

• Herbal soak. Make a strong tea of comfrey and organic goldenseal. Pour the warm tea into a small glass and place the penis in it for as long as possible. (For children, this may be only a few minutes, considering the activity level of most small boys.) As an alternative method, soak a soft cotton cloth in the tea and place it directly on the infected area.

• Herbal wash a wash made of a decoction of witch hazel bark (not the extract), white oak bark, and raspberry leaf. Gently wash the infected area two or three times daily with this astringent, disinfectant tea.

If the infection persists, treat it internally with a mixture of organically grown goldenseal or chaparral, echinacea, marsh mallow root, and myrrh. These herbs can be powdered and encapsulated in size 0 caps and taken at regular intervals throughout the day. Give small children 1 capsule three times daily. For infants, mix a pinch of the powder with warm milk or juice. Adults may take 2 capsules three times daily.

This mixture, useful for many types of infections, can also be tinctured. For a small child or an infant, mix 3 to 10 drops of the tincture in warm water, milk, or tea and administer three times daily. For adults, take ¼ teaspoon of the tincture three to six times daily.

Urinary Tract Infections

Weak bladders and urinary tract infections often plague men, most probably due to the placement of that male organ, the prostate. Drink cranberry juice. Drink 2 to 4 glasses of cranberry juice daily. Cranberries are the natural treatment of choice for the bladder and the kidneys, since they contain a chemical that prevents bacteria from adhering to the urethra wall, thus helping prevent urinary tract infection. If you're prone to bladder infections, keep on hand unsweetened cranberry juice.

Dilute the tart juice with apple juice or tea. You also can use fresh or frozen cranberries and cranberry tablets for urinary tract infections. Use herbs to support the system. There are a host of

wonderful herbs used to support urinary health, including:

• Buchu

• Corn silk

• Couch grass

• Dandelion leaves

• Goldenseal (organically grown)

• Marsh mallow root

• Oregon grape root

• Saw palmetto

• Uva-ursi

Practice kegel exercises. Kegel exercises are the best strengthening tool we have for toning and conditioning the bladder and the entire genitourinary tract. They were designed by a doctor to treat urinary incontinence.

Treating Inguinal Hernia

Though not normally classified as a male health problem, far more men than women get hernias. Hernias often result from heavy lifting or straining or because the tissue or muscle at the lower end of the abdominal cavity is either congenitally weak or becomes weak and loosens, leaving an opening through which a loop of the intestines protrudes. Inguinal hernias are most often noticed as a lump protruding from the lower abdomen and sometimes a pain that radiates from the groin.

The pain can become □uite severe. Chronic constipation can exacerbate inguinal hernias, since the straining will create extra pressure.

To treat a hernia, apply clay packs to the affected area twice daily. Any clay will do, but my preference for medicinal purposes is green volcanic clay. Mix the clay with enough water to form a paste and apply it directly to the hernia. Cover with a cotton cloth and hold in place with a bandage. Hernia supports can be obtained at most medical supply stores. The clay poultice can be wrapped in gauze and placed inside the support belt. Wear this for at least an hour a day, and longer if it's not too uncomfortable. If you suffer from a hernia, avoid all lifting and straining.

Take care to avoid constipation: Drink plenty of water and supplement with gentle herbal bowel tonics, such as psyllium, yellow dock root, and licorice root. If you develop constipation, take small amounts of senna or cascara sagrada blended with fennel and licorice root. In addition, take 2,000 mg of vitamin C daily and drink herb teas that are astringent and healing.

Oatstraw and horsetail hernia remedy

4 parts comfrey leaf (optional)

3 parts raspberry

2 parts lemon balm

2 parts nettle

2 parts white oak bark

1 part horsetail

1 part oatstraw

Make an infusion of the herbs. Drink 3 to 4 cups daily.

Herbs for Heart Health

Hawthorn, in its many delicious forms, is an absolute must. Include it as a food, tea, and medicine (tinctures and capsules) daily. Studies in Europe have verified its ability to reduce angina attacks as well as lower blood pressure and serum cholesterol levels. Hawthorn is a food herb and can be used safely with heart medication.

Other tonic herbs that are specific for heart health are motherwort, garlic, valerian, cayenne, and yarrow. Each of these herbs has a specific toning effect on the heart.

Hypertension

Hypertension, or high blood pressure, is one of the major medical problems of the 21st century. It is directly related to cardiovascular disease, angina, and heart attacks. Although 92 percent of all diagnosed cases of hypertension are termed essential (i.e., the underlying mechanism is unknown), the primary cause is almost always directly related to diet, stress, and lifestyle choices. Hypertension is almost unknown in undeveloped regions of the world where people still enjoy a diet untainted by fast food and other overprocessed culinary wonders of modern civilization. In these regions, hypertension is not a common, accepted aspect of aging, as it is in more developed countries.

Excess body weight, caffeine, alcohol, stress, smoking, and lack of exercise are major factors contributing to hypertension. Given the wide range of side effects — including impotence and exhaustion — attributed to antihypertensive medication, it seems exceptionally worthwhile to consider lifestyle changes related to the above factors as your primary "treatment."

To treat hypertension, consider the following:

Coenzyme Q10 plays a significant role in metabolic processes involved with energy production. Individuals with cardiovascular disease and hypertension show decreased levels of coenzyme Q10. Supplements are available. Essential fatty acids, especially those found in black currant seeds, flaxseed, and evening primrose, have a profound effect on hypertension. Flaxseed can be ground and added to food. (Store it in the refrigerator to reduce rancidity.)

Garlic is very effective for normalizing blood pressure Levels. Encapsulated garlic, which is mostly odorless, also works well. Other helpful herbs are hawthorn, motherwort, onion, shiitake mushroom, Siberian ginseng, vervain, and yarrow.

High-potassium herbs, such as dandelion leaf have a mild diuretic action and work as a kidney tonic as well. The health of the heart is directly connected to the health of the kidneys. Mistletoe is one of the most widely used herbs for hypertension in Europe, where it is frequently combined with hawthorn. However, mistletoe can be very toxic, even in moderate doses. Use only under the supervision of a competent herbalist or naturopathic doctor.

The Art of Making Herbal Remedies

The most common medicinal herb preparations are tinctures, capsules, and teas. But don't limit yourself to these three. Herbs can be prepared and administered in numerous ways, many of which don't necessarily seem like "medicine."

Syrups and elixirs are an incredibly effective way to extract the medicinal properties of herbs, and they're delicious. Add powdered herbs to salads, shakes, hot cereal, stir-fries, soups, and other dishes, or mix the powders into a paste with honey and spices for a delectable daily tonic. Some herbs, such as hawthorn and elder, can be prepared as tasty jams and jellies — not a bad way to take your medicine. Warm baths are one of the most relaxing and enjoyable ways to use herbs. When you soak in a warm herbal bath, the pores of the skin, the largest organ of elimination and assimilation, are wide open and receptive. It's like soaking in a giant cup of tea; your entire body reaps the benefits.

Buying And Storing Herbs

In these times, when wild lands are being developed at an alarming pace and cultivation of medicinal herbs has not yet caught up with the rate of their use, it is critical that each of us takes responsibility for where our herbs are coming from and who is growing and harvesting them. You must insist on high □uality organically grown herbs. Though they may cost a bit

more, they are far better for our medicines and, ultimately, our planet. Make every effort not to use herbs that are endangered or at risk.

If we wish to preserve this system of healing for our children as it has been passed down to us from our ancestors, preservation of medicinal plant species is imperative. You are supporting not only your own health but the health of the planet when you buy organically grown herbs.

Buying High-Quality Herbs

The single most important factor when purchasing herbs for making remedies is recognizing and obtaining the best quality available. Buy your herbs from reputable companies, those that have a conscience and are concerned about both the quality of the products they sell and the environment. Ask where their herbs come from. Are they organically grown? Are they wildcrafted? If so, were they collected ethically, with respect for the environment?

Whenever possible, use your herbs fresh. However, for a variety of reasons, it is not always feasible to obtain fresh herbs. Dried herbs, if harvested and dried properly, will generally retain all of their medicinal properties. How do you tell if a dried herb is of good □uality? It should look, smell, and taste almost exactly as it does when it's fresh, and it should be effective in your herbal remedies.

Storing Herbs

Herbs retain their properties best if stored in airtight glass jars, away from direct light, in a cool storage area. For convenience, you can store them in many other containers — boxes, tins, plastic bags — but most herbalists find that those durable glass bottles work best for storage. Each herb has its own "shelf life," or duration of time in which it remains viable. Following one set rule for assigning "expiration dates" for herbs could mean you would throw out perfectly fine peppermint while using poor-quality chickweed. Instead, use the standards of quality — look, taste, and smell — outlined above to determine if your herbs have retained their quality.

Color

A dried herb should be almost the same color as it is when fresh. Dried quantities of green-leaved plants such as peppermint or spearmint should be vividly green. Blossoms should be bright and colorful. Calendula flowers, for example, should be bright orange or yellow. Roots, though generally very subtly hued to begin with, should remain true to their original color. Goldenseal root should be a golden green, echinacea root a silvery brown, yellow dock root a yellowish brown. You may not always know what the correct color of a plant should be, but look for liveliness, vibrancy, and deep, strong colors. You will soon develop a knack for judging herb supplies by their appearance.

Smell

Herbs have distinctive odors that serve as effective means of determining □uality. They should smell strongly, not necessarily "good." The scent of valerian, for instance, has been likened to that of dirty socks; good-quality valerian should smell like really dirty socks. Good-□uality peppermint will make your nose tingle and your eyes water. Some herbs, such as alfalfa, just smell "green," but in that green odor is a freshness and unmistakable vitality.

Taste

Herbs should have a distinctive fresh flavor. Judge taste on potency rather than flavor.

Growing Your Own Medicinal Herbs

The best way to ensure that you're getting quality herbs is to grow your own. Many of the plants that you use for medicine can be grown as part of your vegetable and flower garden. Incorporate them into your landscape and use them as they grow and thrive. Though many herbs have specific habitats and limited range — which is one reason they are threatened — we are finding that many of them are far more adaptable than was previously thought.

Fresh Versus Dried

There is nothing quite as good as the taste of fresh picked herbs. However, many herbs are not available fresh year-round. Fresh herb blends must be used immediately, of course, while dried mixtures can be stored for several months or longer. You can mix fresh and dried herbs for immediate use. For instance, you can mix fresh peppermint with dried ginger root and cinnamon bark to make a stimulating, refreshing tea.

The Kitchen Lab

A kitchen, with all of its marvelous tools, will supply you with most of the utensils you need for preparing herbal products. One of the few rules that most herbalists agree on is never to use aluminum pans for preparing herbs. Aluminum is a proved toxic substance, and the toxicity is easily released by heat into our food. Use glass, stainless steel, ceramic, cast iron, or enamel cooking equipment.

Some useful items are:

• Canning jars for storing herbs and making tinctures

• Cheesecloth or fine muslin for straining herbs

• Coffee grinder reserved for grinding herbs, not coffee

(else your herbs will taste like coffee and your coffee like herbs)

• Grater reserved for grating beeswax

• Large, double-meshed, stainless-steel strainer

• Measuring cups (though, heaven forbid, I hardly use them)

• Stainless-steel pots with tight-fitting lids

It is wise to assemble all the ingredients and utensils you need ahead of time.

Determining Dosage

Even in conventional allopathic medicine, determination of dosage is far more arbitrary than we're led to believe. Herbalists are usually quicker to admit that determining dosage involves some skill and experience, a healthy touch of "inner knowing," careful observation, and a bit of guesswork. To determine the proper dosage of an herbal preparation, you must consider the herbs used to make it: What are their primary actions? Do they have any toxic side effects? Are they tonic in nature or are they used to treat a specific health problem or organ system? Consider the constitution of the person: Is she or he relatively healthy? Robust or sensitive? Weak or debilitated? And, finally, consider the nature of the imbalance or illness you want to address: Is it chronic or acute? Excess or deficient in nature?

These clinical factors will help you determine a reasonable dosage, but ultimately you must trust the wisdom of your own body (or that of the person being treated). Listen to what it tells you. Watch how it responds. The body itself offers the best guidelines for what — and how much — it needs. For those who are just beginning their herbal studies, the guidelines at right will be helpful in getting started. Remember always to use the smallest dosage that will get the job done, working up only as necessary.

Infusions

Infusions are made from the more delicate parts of the plant, including the leaves, flowers, and aromatic parts. These fragile plant parts must be steeped, rather than simmered, because they give up their medicinal properties more easily than do the tougher roots and barks.

To make an infusion, simply boil 1 quart of water per ounce of herb (or 1 cup of water to 1 tablespoon of herb). Pour water over the herb(s) and let steep for 30 to 60 minutes. The proportion of water to herb and the required time to infuse varies greatly, depending on the herb. Start out with the above proportions and then experiment. The more herb you use and the longer you let it steep, the stronger the brew. Let your taste buds and your senses guide you.

Decoctions

Decoctions are made from the more tenacious parts of the plant, such as the roots, bark, and seeds. It's a little harder to extract the constituents from these parts, so a slow simmer (or an overnight infusion) is often required. To make a decoction, place the herbs in a small saucepan and cover with cold water. Heat slowly and simmer, covered, for 20 to 45 minutes. The longer you simmer the herbs, the stronger the tea will be.

Syrups

Syrups are the yummiest of all herbal preparations. They are delicious, concentrated extracts of the herbs cooked into a sweet medicine with the addition of honey and/or fruit juice. Maple syrup and vegetable glycerin may be substituted for honey.

Step 1. Use 2 ounces of herb mixture to 1 quart of water. Over low heat, simmer the liquid down to 1 pint. This will give you a very concentrated tea.

Step 2. Strain the herbs from the liquid. Pour the liquid back into the pot.

Step 3. To each pint of liquid, add 1 cup of honey (or othersweetener, such as maple syrup, vegetable glycerin, or brown sugar). Most recipes call for 2 cups of sweetener (a 1:1 ratio of sweetener to liquid). I find this far too sweet for my taste, but the added sugar helped preserve the syrup in the days when refrigeration wasn't common.

Step 4. Warm the honey and the liquid together only enough to mix well. Most recipes instruct you to cook the honey and the tea together for 20 to 30 minutes over high heat to thicken further. It certainly does make thicker syrup, but I'd rather not cook the living enzymes out of the honey.

Step 5. When the syrup is thoroughly mixed, you may wish to add a fruit concentrate to flavor, or a couple of drops of essential oil, such as peppermint or spearmint, or a small amount of brandy to help preserve the syrup and to aid as a relaxant in cough formulas.

Step 6. Remove from the heat, bottle, and label. Syrups will last for several weeks, even months, if refrigerated.

Herbal Baths

Herbal baths are deeply relaxing. They help take the edge off the day, calm and quiet the mind, encourage deep sleep, and sometimes are just the comfort one needs in a rough and busy world. And aside from your bed, your bathtub may be the most sensuously arousing place in your home, perhaps yet undiscovered. Several prominent healers administer most of their herbal formulas via the bath.

Depending on the herbs you use and the temperature of the water, you can create a bath that is relaxing, stimulating, uplifting, soothing, decongesting, or otherwise curative. Herbal baths open up the pores of the skin, our largest organ of elimination and assimilation.

Herbal bathing used to be far more popular than it is today. But as with so many other things in our busy lives, efficiency has won out over quietude, and the □uick "in and out" of showers has replaced the slow, peaceful nature of bathing. Perhaps this is simply because modern bathtubs tend to be so small and shallow. A hot herbal bath is definitely not relaxing if half of you is sticking out of the tub, freezing! You might consider investing in an old-style claw foot tub — it's well worth it.

The temperature of the water will affect the healing □uality of the bath. Cool to tepid water is excellent for lowering afever or normalizing the system. A warm bath is relaxing and soothing to the nervous system. Cold water is stimulating and contracting and will firm and strengthen the entire system if you're brave enough to endure it.

To make an herbal bath, use 3 to 4 ounces of herb per tub. Use the herbs to make an extra-strong herbal tea; strain and add the tea to the bathwater. Alternatively, bundle the mixed herbs in a large cotton scarf or clean nylon stocking and tie it directly onto the nozzle of the tub. Run hot water through the herbal bundle until the tub is half filled, then toss the bundle in the tub and adjust the temperature with cold water. Soak in the bath for 20 to 30 minutes to enjoy the full benefits of the herbs.

Hand baths and footbaths are also wonderful ways to take advantage of the healing power of herbs. All of the nerves in the body pass through the feet and the hands, making them a map of our inner being. Simply choose an appropriate sized container and adjust the proportion of herbs to water accordingly.

CONCLUSION

It has often been said that modern medicine, the Western allopathic model so familiar to us today, is a heroic system of medicine. It is the medical model of choice for emergency situations, for the "cut and stitch" care needed in accidents and life-threatening situations. The healer is often the hero. Allopathic medicine offers ☐uick fixes and crisis intervention but does not support a person's natural process of healing and does not encourage preventive health care.

Allopathic and herbal medicine together form a perfect balance for the many health problems facing both men and women today. Men are just discovering the same potential for their own herbal health care that women have been taking advantage of for years. Herbs such as saw palmetto, St.- John's-wort, nettle, and ginseng are finding their way into health care products for men, not as a crisis type of medicine but as preventives. Perhaps as men find ways to explore their own health and healing, they'll have less need for crisis intervention, because they will focus on prevention and wellbeing.

Perhaps we'll find more information readily available on men's herbal health. And perhaps we'll experience a boom in the population of male herbalists.

www.ingramcontent.com/pod-product-compliance
Lightning Source LLC
Chambersburg PA
CBHW050758240726
48654CB00008B/548